# UTIS

# DECODED

## Solutions For a Stress-Free Flow

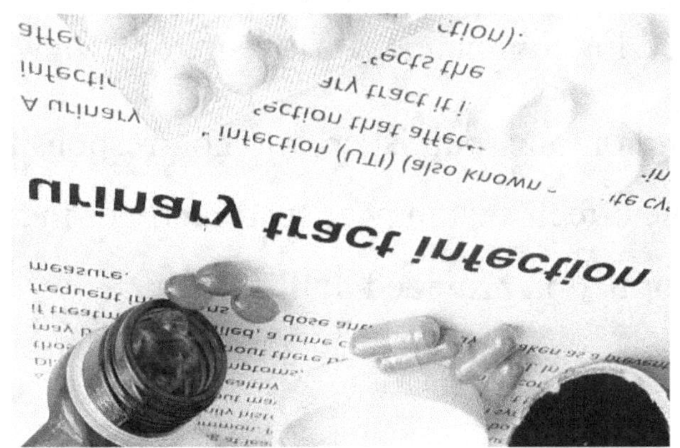

## BROOKLYN LUCAS

This book is designed for educational and informational purposes only. The content aims to enhance understanding and appreciation of health-related topics. Any references to specific events, names, or copyrighted materials are included for commentary, criticism, or review.

The author and publisher are not responsible for any negative effects that may arise, directly or indirectly, from the information provided in this book.

# TABLE OF CONTENT

# INTRODUCTION

The first time it happened, I was young and invincible, at least that's what I thought. A dull ache settled low in my abdomen, a nagging discomfort that escalated into a sharp, burning sensation every time, I used the bathroom. Laughter became a sharp cough, intimacy a distant memory. The constant urge to pee, even after emptying my bladder, was relentless. It was a symphony of discomfort, a constant reminder that something was terribly wrong.

Frustration gnawed at me. I felt blindsided, utterly unprepared for the physical and emotional toll this invisible enemy was taking. Doctor visits, tests, and a course of antibiotics offered temporary relief, but the fear of recurrence loomed large.

This book wasn't born from sterile medical textbooks, but from the very real experience of countless women (and some men) who face the frustration and discomfort of UTIs. It's a story of understanding, of taking control, and of finding ways to navigate a world where a simple bathroom trip can become a battlefield.

In this book, you'll find the knowledge and tools to transform the burning sting of a UTI into a manageable inconvenience. We'll delve into the science behind UTIs, explore effective prevention strategies, and navigate the world of treatment options, both traditional and complementary. Most importantly, we'll empower you to take charge of your urinary health and reclaim a life free from constant worry.

So, join me on this journey of understanding and empowerment. Let's turn that feeling of helplessness into a sense of control. Let's decode UTIs together, and achieve the stress-free flow we all deserve.

# CHAPTER ONE

## 1.1 UNVEILING THE URINARY SYSTEM: A TOUR OF YOUR PIPES

The human body is a marvel of twisted systems working in harmony. One such system, often relegated to the background of our health consciousness, is the urinary tract. This remarkable plumbing network plays a vital role in maintaining our well-being by filtering waste products from the blood and eliminating them from the body. Yet, when a UTI disrupts this efficient system, the once-mysterious urinary tract comes sharply into focus.

Understanding the anatomy of the urinary tract is the first step towards conquering UTIs. Think of it as a fascinating production line, each component contributing to the smooth flow of waste removal. Let's embark on a guided tour and meet the key players in this internal filtration system:

## The Powerhouse Duo: The Kidneys

Picture two bean-shaped marvels perched just above your waist – these are your kidneys.  Don't be fooled by their unassuming size; these powerhouses are constantly working overtime. They act as the body's natural filtration units, meticulously sifting through your blood to remove waste products, excess water, and toxins. The leftover liquid waste becomes urine, a clear yellowish fluid that carries these unwanted substances away.

## The Speedy Couriers: The Ureters

Once the kidneys have created urine, it needs a way to travel. Enter the ureters, a pair of slender tubes that act as the couriers in this system.  Imagine two thin highways, each about the width of a shoelace, extending from the kidneys down to the bladder.  These muscular tubes are lined with smooth muscle cells that contract in a wave-like motion, propelling urine downwards in a one-way journey.

**The Holding Tank: The Bladder**

The next stop on our tour is the bladder, a muscular sac located in the lower abdomen. Think of it as a temporary storage reservoir for urine. As urine trickles down from the ureters, the bladder fills up like a balloon. The bladder wall is made up of smooth muscle that stretches and relaxes to accommodate increasing urine volume. Nerve endings in the bladder wall send signals to the brain when it's time to empty the tank, triggering the familiar urge to urinate.

**The Final Exit Point: The Urethra**

The final leg of the urinary tract journey takes place through the urethra, a narrow tube that acts as the exit point for urine. Imagine a short straw extending from the base of the bladder and leading out of the body. The urethra is lined with a special type of tissue that helps prevent urine from leaking back up into the bladder. When we urinate, the bladder muscles contract, while the sphincter muscles surrounding the urethra relax, allowing urine to flow out of the body.

## Nerves and Muscles Working Together

While the organs themselves are crucial, the urinary tract relies on a delicate ballet of nerves and muscles to function smoothly. Nerves in the bladder wall constantly monitor urine volume, sending signals to the brain when it's time to empty. The brain then sends messages back to the bladder and urethra, coordinating the muscle contractions that allow for urine storage and release.

The ureters, for instance, utilize smooth muscle contractions to propel urine downwards in a peristaltic wave. Think of a wave rolling through a crowd, pushing people forward. Similarly, these contractions create a wave-like motion that effectively pushes urine down the ureters towards the bladder.

## Maintaining the Balance: The Body's Natural Defenses

The urinary tract may seem like a simple plumbing network, but it's a highly evolved system with built-in defenses. The lining of the urinary tract acts as a barrier against infection. This lining secretes mucus, which acts like a sticky flypaper, trapping and preventing bacteria from adhering to the walls and establishing an infection.

Another crucial defense mechanism is the constant flow of urine. Think of it as a natural flush system. By regularly emptying the bladder, we help wash away bacteria that might try to gain a foothold in the urinary tract. Staying hydrated ensures sufficient urine volume to effectively flush out potential invaders.

Finally, the urogenital area harbors a delicate balance of microbial flora. These "good" bacteria help prevent the overgrowth of harmful bacteria that could lead to a UTI. Think of them as friendly guards that keep unwanted visitors at bay.

**Understanding the Anatomy: The Key to Prevention**

By understanding the anatomy of the urinary tract, we gain valuable insights into how UTIs occur. Knowing the different components and their functions allows us to identify potential weaknesses and adopt preventive measures. For instance, staying hydrated ensures sufficient urine flow to flush out bacteria, while maintaining proper hygiene practices helps prevent bacteria from entering the urethra.

Furthermore, understanding the delicate balance of the urogenital flora allows us to make informed decisions about products we use in that area, minimizing disruption to the natural bacterial community. The more we know about the twisted. workings of the urinary tract, the better equipped we are to maintain its health and prevent UTIs.

**Additional Players in the System**

While the kidneys, ureters, bladder, and urethra are the core components of the urinary tract, there are other players that contribute to its overall function:

Sphincters: These are muscular rings that act as valves, controlling the flow of urine. Two sphincters play a vital role: the internal urethral sphincter, located at the base of the bladder, and the external urethral sphincter, located just below it. The internal sphincter is an involuntary muscle, while the external sphincter can be controlled consciously.

The coordinated action of these sphincters allows us to store urine until we can reach a restroom and urinate voluntarily.

Pelvic Floor Muscles: These muscles form a hammock-like structure that supports the bladder, uterus (in females), and rectum. Strong pelvic floor muscles contribute to urinary control by helping to maintain continence and prevent involuntary leakage.

**The Importance of Maintaining Urinary Tract Health**

The urinary tract is a remarkable system that works tirelessly behind the scenes to maintain our health. By understanding its anatomy and the delicate balance that keeps it functioning smoothly, we can take proactive steps towards preventing UTIs. Simple lifestyle modifications, such as staying hydrated, maintaining proper hygiene, and strengthening pelvic floor muscles, can significantly reduce the risk of infection.

Remember, the more we know about the urinary tract, the more empowered we become to take charge of our health and achieve a stress-free flow.  The remaining chapters of this book will sift deeper into the causes and symptoms of UTIs, explore effective prevention strategies, and navigate the world of treatment options.  Together, we can turn the tide on UTIs and reclaim control of our urinary health.

## 1.2 The Troublemakers: Bacteria and Their UTI Games

While the urinary tract boasts impressive defenses, it's not invincible.  Urinary tract infections (UTIs) occur when bacteria manage to infiltrate this well-guarded system, causing inflammation and discomfort.  Understanding the different types of bacteria that cause UTIs and their sneaky tactics of invasion is crucial for effective prevention.

### E. coli: The Notorious Neighbor

The most common culprit behind UTIs is a familiar foe – Escherichia coli, or E. coli for short.  This bacterium is a natural resident of our intestines, aiding in digestion by breaking down food.  However, E. coli can become a villain when it ventures beyond its designated territory.

The short distance between the urethra and the anus makes it all too easy for E. coli to make a wrong turn. Improper wiping techniques, from back to front instead of front to back, can inadvertently transfer E. coli from the anus to the urethra, creating a prime opportunity for infection.

**Beyond E. coli: Other Bacterial Troublemakers**

While E. coli takes the top spot, other types of bacteria can also cause UTIs. Here are some of the less frequent offenders:

1. Staphylococcus saprophyticus: This bacterium is commonly found on the skin and can sometimes find its way into the urethra, particularly in young, sexually active women.

2. Klebsiella pneumoniae: This bacterium is part of the normal gut flora, but it can occasionally cause UTIs, especially in individuals with weakened immune systems or those who have undergone urinary tract procedures involving catheters.

3. Enterococcus faecalis: This bacterium is another resident of the intestines and can sometimes cause UTIs, particularly in healthcare settings or in individuals with recurrent UTIs.

## The Invasion Routes: How Bacteria Breach the Defenses

Once bacteria like E. coli find themselves near the urethral opening, they need a way to penetrate the urinary tract defenses. Here's how these sneaky invaders might gain a foothold:

1. Ascending the Stream: The most common route of invasion involves bacteria ascending the urethra and traveling upwards towards the bladder. Factors that disrupt the natural flow of urine, such as infrequent urination or incomplete bladder emptying, can create an environment where bacteria have more time to linger and multiply.

2. Catheter Complications: Urinary catheters, inserted into the bladder to drain urine, can provide a direct pathway for bacteria to enter the urinary tract, especially if proper

sterile procedures are not followed during catheter insertion and maintenance.

3. Sexual Activity: Sexual intercourse can introduce bacteria from the vagina or rectum into the urethra, particularly if proper hygiene practices aren't followed before and after sex. Certain sexual practices, like using spermicides, can also disrupt the balance of vaginal flora, increasing the risk of UTIs.

4. Underlying Abnormalities: Structural abnormalities in the urinary tract, such as a blockage in the urethra or a malfunctioning urethral sphincter, can create stagnant urine pools where bacteria can thrive. These conditions can make UTIs more recurrent.

**Understanding Risk Factors: Who's More Susceptible?**

Certain factors can increase your susceptibility to UTIs by creating conditions that favor bacterial growth or hindering the body's natural defenses. Here are some risk factors to be aware of:

- Gender: Women have a shorter urethra compared to men, making it easier for bacteria to travel from the urethra to the bladder. Additionally, hormonal changes during pregnancy and menopause can affect the vaginal flora, increasing the risk of UTIs.

- Sexual Activity: Sexually active women are more prone to UTIs, particularly after intercourse. Frequent use of spermicides can also disrupt the vaginal flora, further increasing susceptibility.

- Urinary Tract Issues: Conditions like bladder prolapse, which weakens the pelvic floor muscles, or kidney stones, which can obstruct urine flow, can create an environment conducive to UTIs.

- Catheter Use: Individuals who rely on catheters for urinary drainage are at a higher risk of UTIs due to the direct access these devices provide for bacteria to enter the bladder.

- Impaired Immunity: Conditions that weaken the immune system, such as diabetes or HIV/AIDS, can make individuals more susceptible to UTIs.

- Personal Hygiene: Poor hygiene practices, such as infrequent urination or improper wiping techniques, can increase the risk of bacteria entering the urethra.

- Knowledge is Power: Taking Control of Your Urinary Health

By understanding the different types of bacteria that cause UTIs and the various ways they infiltrate the urinary tract, we gain valuable knowledge for prevention. Simple lifestyle modifications, such as maintaining good hygiene practices, staying hydrated to promote regular urination, and emptying your bladder completely after urination, can significantly reduce your risk of UTIs.

# CHAPTER TWO

## 2.1 BEYOND THE BURN: A RANGE OF UTI SIGNS

Urinary tract infections (UTIs) are notorious for the burning sensation they unleash, making bathroom trips a battlefield. However, UTIs can manifest in a variety of ways, and the discomfort isn't always the most obvious sign. Recognizing the spectrum of UTI symptoms empowers you to seek timely diagnosis and treatment, restoring a stress-free flow to your life.

### The Discomfort Duo: Burning and Frequency

The classic UTI duo – burning urination (dysuria) and frequent urination (urinary urgency) – are often the first signs that trouble is brewing in your urinary tract. The burning sensation, often described as a stinging or itching, occurs when the inflamed lining of the urethra comes into contact with urine. Urinary urgency, the persistent urge to urinate even after passing a small amount of urine, can be relentless and disruptive.

## Beyond the Basics: Less Common Symptoms

While the burning and frequency duo are the most recognized UTI symptoms, several other signs can indicate a brewing infection. Here's a broader range of symptoms to be aware of:

Pelvic Pain: A dull ache or pressure in the lower abdomen, particularly around the pubic bone, can be a symptom of a UTI. This discomfort can be intensified with urination.

Hematuria (Blood in Urine): The presence of blood in urine, even in small amounts, can be a sign of a UTI, particularly if accompanied by other symptoms. It's important to note that blood in urine can also be caused by other conditions, so seeking medical attention is crucial.

Cloudy or Foul-Smelling Urine: Healthy urine is typically clear or pale yellow with a mild odor. However, a UTI can cause urine to become cloudy or develop a strong ammonia-like smell.

Urinary Incontinence: The inability to control urination, leading to involuntary leakage, can be a symptom of a UTI, especially in older adults. This is more likely if the infection reaches the kidneys and causes inflammation.

Flank Pain: In severe UTIs, particularly those affecting the kidneys (pyelonephritis), a sharp pain may be felt on one or both sides of the lower back, near the ribs. This is due to inflammation of the kidneys.

Fever and Chills: A low-grade fever and chills can sometimes accompany a UTI, particularly if the infection spreads to the kidneys.

**Variations in Presentation: Understanding Differences**

It's important to note that UTI symptoms can vary depending on the location of the infection. Here's a breakdown of how symptoms might differ:

Urethritis: This infection affects the urethra, the tube that carries urine out of the body. Burning urination and frequent urination are the most common symptoms.

Cystitis: This is the most common type of UTI, affecting the bladder. In addition to burning and frequency, you might experience pelvic pain or blood in the urine.

Pyelonephritis: This infection reaches the kidneys, causing the most severe symptoms, including flank pain, fever, chills, and nausea in addition to the usual burning and frequency.

**Don't Ignore the Signs:  Seeking Timely Diagnosis**

While the symptoms described above can be indicative of a UTI, it's crucial to remember that other conditions may mimic these signs. Delaying diagnosis and treatment can worsen the infection and lead to complications.  Therefore, if you experience any combination of these symptoms, particularly if they persist for more than a day or two, it's vital to consult with your doctor.

Through a simple urine test, your doctor can confirm the presence of bacteria and determine the specific type of UTI you have. Early diagnosis and appropriate treatment are key to a speedy recovery and preventing complications.

The next section of this book will go into the reasons why UTIs occur. We'll explore how bacteria manage to infiltrate the urinary tract defenses and the various factors that can increase your susceptibility to these infections. Equipped with this knowledge, we can embark on a journey of effective prevention and maintain a healthy, well-functioning urinary tract.

## 2.2 When to Seek Help: Differentiating UTIs from Other Issues

Urinary tract infections (UTIs) can be a real party crasher, turning a simple bathroom trip into a battlefield. However, the discomfort and urgency they cause can sometimes mimic symptoms of other conditions. Vaginal infections, bladder issues, and even sexually transmitted infections (STIs) can wear similar disguises, making it a challenge to identify the true culprit. Fear not, for this chapter equips you with detective skills to differentiate UTIs from these imposters, ensuring you get the right diagnosis and treatment for a speedy recovery.

**The Burning Question: UTIs vs. Bladder Infections**

The terms "UTI" and "bladder infection" are often used interchangeably, and for good reason. Cystitis, the most common type of UTI, affects the bladder, so the symptoms can appear quite similar. Here's how to distinguish between the two:

Symptoms Beyond Burning: While both UTIs and bladder infections can cause burning urination and frequent urination, UTIs are more likely to present with additional symptoms like pelvic pain, blood in the urine, and a strong urine odor. Bladder infections, on the other hand, might cause vaginal discharge or discomfort during sex, which are not typical UTI symptoms.

The Culprit: UTIs are caused by bacteria entering the urinary tract, while bladder infections can have a different origin. Interstitial cystitis (IC), for instance, is a chronic bladder condition that causes pain, pressure, and urgency without the presence of bacteria.

Seeking the Truth: A urine test is your best friend in this detective work. This simple test can reveal the presence of bacteria, a hallmark of UTIs, and help differentiate it from other bladder issues. Additionally, your doctor might perform a pelvic exam to check for signs of vaginal infections or other underlying conditions.

## The STI Imposter: When UTIs Mimic Sexually Transmitted Infections

Certain sexually transmitted infections (STIs) can also masquerade as UTIs, further complicating the diagnosis. Here's how to tell them apart:

The Discharge Dilemma: While UTIs can sometimes cause a slight vaginal discharge, it's not a typical symptom. STIs like gonorrhea or chlamydia, on the other hand, often present with abnormal vaginal discharge, along with burning urination and pelvic pain.

Beyond the Urinary Tract: STIs can affect other areas of the reproductive system, causing symptoms like vaginal itching, burning during sex, and even cervical pain. UTIs, on the other hand, primarily affect the urinary tract and typically don't cause these additional symptoms.

Partner in Diagnosis: If you're sexually active and experiencing UTI-like symptoms, it's crucial to inform your doctor. They might recommend additional tests for STIs to ensure a comprehensive diagnosis.

## When the Lines Blur: Overlapping Symptoms and the Importance of Diagnosis

It's important to acknowledge that there can be some overlap in symptoms between UTIs, bladder infections, and STIs. For instance, some STIs, like chlamydia, can cause burning urination without necessarily causing a noticeable discharge.

Therefore, relying solely on symptoms for diagnosis is risky. If you experience any combination of these symptoms, particularly if they persist for more than a day or two, it's vital to consult your doctor. A urine test and potentially other examinations, depending on your specific situation, will help your doctor differentiate between UTIs and other conditions, ensuring you receive the most appropriate treatment.

## The Importance of Early Intervention

Early diagnosis and treatment are crucial for any infection, but especially for UTIs. Left untreated, UTIs can ascend the urinary tract and reach the kidneys, leading to a more serious condition called pyelonephritis. This can cause severe pain, fever, and even permanent kidney damage.

## Know Your Body, Seek Help:

The more you understand your body's normal urinary habits, the easier it becomes to identify when something feels off. Burning urination, frequent urination, pelvic pain, or any other unusual urinary symptoms are a sign to listen to your body and seek medical attention. With a clear diagnosis and appropriate treatment, you can overcome the UTI imposter and reclaim a stress-free flow.

# CHAPTER THREE

## 3.1 HOW WATER FLUSHES OUT TROUBLE

**H2O: Your Superhero Ally in the Fight Against UTIs**

Did you know that staying hydrated is one of the simplest yet most effective ways to prevent urinary tract infections (UTIs)? Think of water as your superhero ally, flushing out bacteria and keeping your urinary tract healthy. But let's face it, keeping up with water intake can feel like a daily battle against forgetfulness and the lure of sugary drinks. Fear not, for this chapter equips you with practical tips and strategies to transform yourself into a hydration hero, effectively conquering UTIs and achieving a healthier you.

**Why Hydration Matters:  The Power of Dilution**

Water is the lifeblood of our bodies, playing a crucial role in numerous functions. When it comes to UTIs, staying hydrated helps dilute urine, preventing bacteria from adhering to the walls of the bladder and urethra. Think of it like washing away unwanted visitors before they have a chance to set up camp and cause an infection.

Dehydration, on the other hand, concentrates urine, creating a breeding ground for bacteria. This concentrated urine can also irritate the bladder lining, leading to discomfort and potentially increasing your susceptibility to UTIs.

**How Much Liquid Do You Need?  The Personalized Approach**

The age-old question of "eight glasses a day" might be a good starting point, but individual needs can vary. Factors like activity level, climate, and overall health can influence how much water your body requires. Here are some personalized approaches to determine your ideal fluid intake:

Listen to Your Body: Thirst is a natural indicator of dehydration. However, waiting until you're parched isn't ideal. Aim to drink fluids throughout the day, even if you don't feel acutely thirsty.

Monitor Your Urine Color: Your urine is a handy biofeedback tool. Strive for pale yellow urine, which indicates proper hydration. Dark yellow or amber-colored urine suggests dehydration.

Factor in Activity Level: Do you break a sweat during exercise? If so, you'll need to replenish fluids lost through perspiration. Increase your water intake before, during, and after workouts.

Consider Your Climate: Hot and humid environments can accelerate dehydration. Living in a tropical paradise or sweating it out during summer months necessitates increased water intake.

**Beyond Water:  Hydration Heroes in Disguise**

While water is the ultimate hydration champion, there are other ways to keep your body's fluid levels in check. Here are some surprise heroes in the hydration game:

Fruits and Vegetables: Many fruits and vegetables boast high water content. Think watermelon, cucumber, celery, and leafy greens. Adding these to your diet provides a refreshing and hydrating boost.

Herbal Teas: Herbal teas, like chamomile or peppermint, are a delightful way to increase fluid intake. Just be mindful of herbal teas with diuretic properties, as they can actually increase urine output and potentially dehydrate you.

Low-Fat Soups: Warm or chilled low-fat soups can be a surprisingly hydrating option. They provide fluids and essential nutrients, adding variety to your hydration routine.

**Transforming into a Hydration Hero: Practical Tips and Strategies**

Conquering UTIs through hydration requires a strategic approach. Here are some practical tips to transform yourself into a hydration hero:

Invest in a Reusable Water Bottle: Carry a reusable water bottle with you throughout the day. Having it readily available serves as a constant reminder to sip and stay hydrated. Choose a bottle you love – a fun design or motivational quote can make it more appealing to reach for.

Set Hydration Reminders: Let technology be your friend. Set phone alerts or use a hydration app to remind yourself to take regular sips throughout the day.

Infuse Your Water: Plain water can sometimes feel monotonous. Jazz it up with slices of cucumber, lemon, or berries for a refreshing twist. Experiment with different flavor combinations to keep things interesting.

Make Water a Habit: Integrate water into your daily routine. Start your day with a glass of water, set a glass beside your meals, and make it a point to drink before bed. The more you automate these habits, the easier it becomes to stay hydrated.

Celebrate Your Success: Track your progress! There are many water tracking apps available to help you monitor your daily intake. Reaching your hydration goals deserves a pat on the back. Celebrate your success and stay motivated to maintain this healthy habit.

**Beyond Hydration:  A Multifaceted Approach to UTI Prevention**

While staying hydrated is a powerful tool in the fight against UTIs, it's not the only weapon in your arsenal.  The following chapters of this book will explore other preventive strategies, such as proper hygiene practices, maintaining pelvic floor strength, and cranberry consumption.  By adopting a multifaceted approach, you can significantly reduce your risk of UTIs and enjoy a healthier urinary tract.

## Waging War on Bacteria:   The Power of Proper Hygiene

Our daily hygiene practices play a vital role in preventing bacteria from entering the urethra and causing UTIs.  Here are some key hygiene tips to remember:

Wipe Front to Back: After using the toilet, always wipe from front to back to prevent bacteria from the anal area from contaminating the urethra.

Urinate After Sex: Sexual activity can introduce bacteria near the urethral opening. Flushing the urinary tract by emptying your bladder soon after sex can help wash away any unwanted visitors.

Avoid Harsh Soaps: Douching or using harsh soaps in the genital area can disrupt the natural balance of vaginal flora, potentially increasing UTI risk. Opt for gentle, fragrance-free cleansers specifically designed for the sensitive genital area.

Cotton is King: Tight-fitting, synthetic underwear can trap moisture and create a breeding ground for bacteria.

Choose loose-fitting, breathable cotton underwear to promote airflow and prevent bacterial growth.

**Building a Strong Defense: The Importance of Pelvic Floor Strength**

The pelvic floor muscles act like a hammock, supporting the bladder, uterus, and rectum. Strong pelvic floor muscles can help improve urinary control and prevent leakage. Here's how strengthening these muscles can benefit your fight against UTIs:

Improved Bladder Control: Strong pelvic floor muscles allow for better closure of the urethra, reducing the risk of urine leakage and potentially preventing bacteria from entering the bladder.

Enhanced Emptying: Pelvic floor exercises can help ensure complete emptying of the bladder, preventing stagnant urine that could harbor bacteria.

There are various pelvic floor exercises, also known as Kegels, that can be easily incorporated into your daily routine. These exercises involve contracting and relaxing the pelvic floor muscles, similar to the sensation of stopping urination midstream. By consistently performing Kegels, you can strengthen these muscles and contribute to a healthier urinary tract.

**A Natural Ally?  Exploring the Role of Cranberries**

Cranberries have long been touted as a natural remedy for UTIs.  Cranberry juice contains certain compounds called proanthocyanidins (PACs) that may prevent bacteria from adhering to the bladder wall.  However, the research on cranberry's effectiveness is somewhat mixed.

While some studies suggest that cranberry juice or cranberry supplements might offer some preventive benefit, particularly for women with recurrent UTIs, the evidence isn't conclusive.  It's important to speak with your doctor to determine if cranberry products might be a suitable addition to your UTI prevention strategy.

**Taking Control of Your Urinary Health**

By understanding the various ways to prevent UTIs, you become an active participant in safeguarding your urinary health. From staying hydrated and maintaining proper hygiene to considering pelvic floor exercises and exploring options like cranberry products, you have a toolkit at your disposal to keep UTIs at bay.

## 3.2 Dehydration's Downside: Making You More Susceptible

We all know the importance of water. It quenches our thirst, regulates our body temperature, and keeps our organs functioning optimally. But did you know that dehydration can be a major contributing factor to urinary tract infections (UTIs)? Think of your body as a well-oiled machine, and water is the essential lubricant. When the lubrication runs low, friction increases, and the machine starts to sputter. In the case of your urinary tract, dehydration creates an environment ripe for UTIs to flourish.

### The Numbers Don't Lie: Dehydration and UTI Risk

Studies have shown a clear link between dehydration and an increased risk of UTIs. A 2016 study published in the journal "Urology" found that women who consumed less fluid were more likely to experience UTIs compared to those who maintained adequate hydration. Another study, published in the "Canadian Journal of Urology" in 2017, showed that increased fluid intake significantly reduced the risk of recurrent UTIs in women.

These numbers paint a clear picture: dehydration isn't just an inconvenience; it can be a recipe for UTIs. Let's explore the specific ways dehydration creates a breeding ground for these pesky infections.

## The Domino Effect of Dehydration: From Concentrated Urine to UTI Havoc

Here's how dehydration sets the stage for UTIs:

Concentrated Trouble: When you don't drink enough fluids, your urine becomes more concentrated. Think of it like a thick syrup compared to a refreshing glass of water. This concentrated urine creates a breeding ground for bacteria, as it provides them with a more favorable environment to multiply.

Flushing Away the Good Guys: Adequate hydration helps flush out bacteria from the urinary tract through urination. Think of it like a natural internal irrigation system. Dehydration reduces urine output, hindering this flushing mechanism and allowing bacteria to linger and potentially establish an infection.

Irritated and Vulnerable: Dehydration can irritate the lining of the bladder. This irritated lining becomes more susceptible to invasion by bacteria, further increasing the risk of a UTI.

**Beyond UTIs: The Ripple Effect of Dehydration**

It's important to remember that UTIs are just one consequence of dehydration. When your body is dehydrated, it can experience a cascade of negative effects, impacting everything from your energy levels and cognitive function to your digestion and immune system.

By staying hydrated, you're not just protecting yourself from UTIs; you're investing in your overall health and well-being.

## Dehydration Disguised

Dehydration doesn't always announce itself with intense thirst.  Here are some subtle signs that you might be dehydrated:

- Fatigue: Feeling sluggish and lacking energy can be a sign that your body is craving fluids.

- Headaches: Dehydration can lead to headaches, making it a double whammy – you not only feel drained, but you might also experience a throbbing head.

- Dry Mouth and Skin: These are classic signs of dehydration. A parched mouth and dry, flaky skin indicate that your body needs more fluids.

- Decreased Urination: If you're not urinating frequently and your urine is dark yellow, it's a strong indicator that you're dehydrated.

## Prioritize Hydration for a Healthy You

Dehydration is a preventable risk factor for UTIs.  By making conscious efforts to stay hydrated throughout the day, you can significantly reduce your susceptibility to these infections. Remember, small changes in your daily routine can have a big impact on your urinary health and overall well-being. So, grab your water bottle, and let's embark on a journey towards optimal hydration and a UTI-free future!

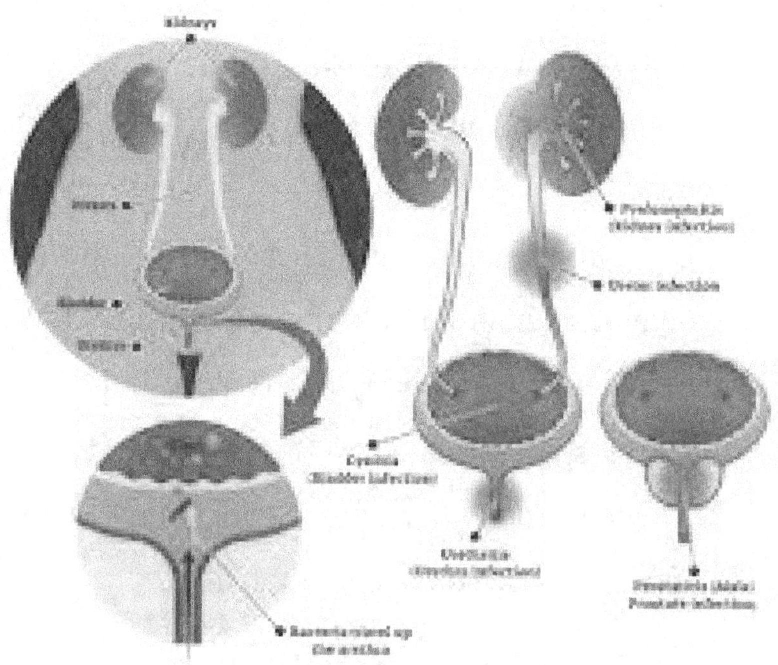

# CHAPTER FOUR

## 4.1 WIPING WISDOM: FRONT TO BACK MATTERS

When it comes to bathroom etiquette, wiping technique might not be the most glamorous topic, but it holds surprising importance in the realm of urinary tract infections (UTIs).  For women, the simple act of wiping can be the difference between a healthy urinary tract and a battle against a bacterial invasion.  This chapter dig into the science behind wiping and unveils why the "front-to-back" method reigns supreme in the fight against UTIs.

### The E. coli Trojan Horse:  Understanding the Threat

Escherichia coli, or E. coli for short, is a bacterium that naturally resides in our intestines.  While some strains are harmless, others can be real troublemakers, particularly for the urinary tract.  E. coli can hitch a ride from the anus to the urethra, the opening of the urinary tract, if proper wiping technique isn't followed.

The short distance between the anus and the urethra creates a vulnerability. Wiping from back to front increases the risk of transferring E. coli from the anal area to the urethra, creating a potential pathway for infection. Think of it like an unwelcome Trojan Horse, sneaking into the urinary tract and wreaking havoc.

**Front to Back: The Wiping Maneuver for UTI Prevention**

The "front-to-back" wiping technique is the undisputed champion in preventing UTIs. Here's why this method is so effective:

Minimizing Bacterial Transfer: By wiping from front to back, you move away from the urethra, minimizing the chances of transferring E. coli or other bacteria from the anus to the urinary tract opening.

Creating a Barrier: Wiping from front to back creates a clean barrier, preventing bacteria from traveling back towards the urethra.

Maintaining Hygiene: This method ensures proper hygiene for both the anal and genital areas, reducing the overall bacterial load in the region.

**Wiping Wisdom for Optimal Hygiene**

Here are some additional tips to elevate your wiping game and further reduce UTI risk:

Use Soft, Fragrance-Free Wipes: Harsh toilet paper or wipes with perfumes can irritate the delicate genital area. Opt for gentle, fragrance-free products that cleanse effectively without causing discomfort.

Double Wiping (if needed): For a thorough clean, especially during menstruation, you might consider wiping twice, once from front to back for the genital area and another from front to back for the anal area, using separate wipes for each.

Cleanliness is Key: Always wash your hands thoroughly with soap and water after using the toilet. This simple step helps prevent the spread of bacteria to other parts of your body.

**Making it a Habit:  The Power of Routine**

While the "front-to-back" technique might seem straightforward, it can take some conscious effort to make it a habit, especially if you've been wiping differently for years.  Here are some strategies to solidify this UTI-fighting behavior:

Visual Reminders: Place a sticky note or label in your bathroom as a visual reminder of the proper wiping direction.

Positive Reinforcement:  Celebrate your progress! Acknowledge your commitment to good hygiene and the positive impact it has on your urinary health.

Educate Others: Share this knowledge with your friends, family members, and even your daughters as they reach puberty. Spreading awareness about proper wiping technique can benefit everyone.

**Small Change, Big Impact**

Taking the time to wipe properly might seem like a minor detail, but when it comes to UTIs, it can make a world of difference. By adopting the "front-to-back" wiping technique, you're taking a proactive step towards preventing these infections and maintaining a healthy urinary tract. So, embrace the "front-to-back" method, and embark on a journey towards a stress-free flow!

## 4.2 Emptying Completely: Don't Hold It In!

We've all been there – the urge to use the bathroom hits, but you're busy, caught up in a conversation, or simply don't feel like interrupting your flow (of activity, that is). However, this seemingly harmless act of holding in your urine can have unintended consequences, particularly when it comes to urinary tract infections (UTIs). This chapter jump into the importance of complete bladder emptying and unveils why resisting the urge to hold back is a winning strategy for UTI prevention.

## The Bladder's Reservoir

The bladder acts as a storage tank for urine, expanding and contracting as needed. While there's no single "ideal" bladder capacity, a healthy adult bladder can typically hold around 16 to 20 ounces of urine. However, exceeding this capacity or frequently holding urine for extended periods can create an environment ripe for UTIs.

## Stagnant Waters, Breeding Grounds for Trouble

When urine remains in the bladder for too long, it becomes stagnant. This stagnant urine provides a breeding ground for bacteria, particularly E. coli, the same culprit often implicated in UTIs. Think of it like a stagnant pond compared to a flowing river. The stagnant pond allows for unchecked bacterial growth, while the flowing river naturally flushes out bacteria.

## Incomplete Emptying: A Double Whammy for UTIs

Holding urine back can also lead to incomplete emptying of the bladder. Residual urine left behind in the bladder creates a double whammy effect for UTIs:

Bacterial Feast: The leftover urine provides a feast for bacteria, allowing them to multiply and potentially cause an infection.

Irritation and Vulnerability: A full bladder can irritate the bladder lining, making it more susceptible to bacterial invasion. Think of it like irritated skin that's more prone to infection.

**The Power of the Flush: Benefits of Complete Emptying**

By completely emptying your bladder whenever you feel the urge to urinate, you're essentially performing a natural internal flush. Here's how this benefits your fight against UTIs:

Reduced Bacterial Growth: Regular emptying prevents urine from becoming stagnant, minimizing the opportunity for bacteria to multiply.

Flushing Out the Troublemakers: Complete emptying helps flush out bacteria that might have entered the bladder, preventing them from establishing an infection.

Maintaining a Healthy Bladder Lining: Regular emptying reduces pressure on the bladder and helps maintain the integrity of the bladder lining, making it less susceptible to irritation and infection.

**Listen to Your Body:  The Urge is Your Guide**

Your body is remarkably good at communicating its needs. The urge to urinate is a natural signal from your body that your bladder is full and needs to be emptied.  Ignoring this urge can disrupt this communication system and lead to problems like UTIs.

**Building the Habit:  Respond to the Urge Promptly**

Making complete bladder emptying a habit might require some practice, especially if you've been conditioned to hold it in for various reasons.  Here are some tips to help you establish this UTI-fighting behavior:

Schedule Bathroom Breaks: Even if you don't feel a strong urge, try to use the restroom every two to four hours. This helps prevent the bladder from becoming overly full.

Relax and Take Your Time: Sometimes, rushing during urination can lead to incomplete emptying. Relax and take your time to allow for complete bladder voiding.

Pelvic Floor Muscle Exercises: Strengthening your pelvic floor muscles can improve bladder control and emptying efficiency. Consider incorporating Kegel exercises into your daily routine.

**Emptying Regularly, a UTI Defense Strategy**

Complete bladder emptying is a simple yet powerful strategy for preventing UTIs. By listening to your body's cues and responding to the urge to urinate promptly, you can help keep your urinary tract healthy and UTI-free. So, ditch the habit of holding back and embrace the power of complete bladder emptying for a healthier you!

# CHAPTER FIVE

## 5.1 CRANBERRY POWERHOUSE: FACT OR FICTION?

Cranberries – those ruby red jewels of the bog – have long been touted as a natural remedy for urinary tract infections (UTIs). For generations, grandmothers have sworn by cranberry juice or cranberry supplements to ward off these pesky infections. But does science back up this age-old tradition? This chapter dives into the research surrounding cranberries and UTIs, separating fact from folklore and helping you understand the potential role these tart berries might play in your UTI prevention strategy.

### The Cranberry Craze: A History of Folk Wisdom

The use of cranberries for urinary health dates back centuries. Native American tribes traditionally used cranberries for various medicinal purposes, including treating bladder ailments. This folk wisdom eventually trickled down through generations, solidifying the cranberry's reputation as a UTI fighter.

## The Science of Proanthocyanidins (PACs): Cranberry's Potential Weapon

So, what's the science behind this cranberry craze? Cranberries are rich in compounds called proanthocyanidins (PACs). These PACs are thought to work in a specific way to potentially prevent UTIs:

Blocking Bacterial Adhesion: Some studies suggest that PACs can prevent E. coli, the common culprit in UTIs, from adhering to the walls of the bladder. Think of it like coating the bladder lining with a slippery shield, making it difficult for bacteria to gain a foothold.

## A Mixed Bag of Results

While the theory behind PACs sounds promising, the research on cranberries and UTIs isn't entirely conclusive. Here's a closer look at the current scientific landscape:

Supportive Studies: Several studies have shown that cranberry juice or cranberry supplements might offer some preventive benefit, particularly for women with recurrent UTIs. These studies suggest that regular cranberry consumption could lead to a decrease in the frequency of UTIs.

Uncertain Impact: Other studies haven't found a significant effect of cranberries on UTI prevention. These studies highlight the need for further research to solidify the potential benefits of cranberries.

**Factors at Play:  The Cranberry Conundrum**

The seemingly conflicting research on cranberries can be attributed to several factors:

Type of Cranberry Product: The effectiveness might vary depending on the type of cranberry product used (juice, capsules, extracts) and the concentration of PACs.

Individual Differences: People may respond differently to cranberry products based on factors like their overall health and susceptibility to UTIs.

Study Design Limitations: Some studies might have limitations in their design or methodology, making it difficult to draw definitive conclusions.

**The Cranberry Conundrum: To Juice or Not to Juice?**

With the current research landscape, it's difficult to make a definitive statement about cranberries as a guaranteed UTI prevention strategy. Here's how to navigate this cranberry conundrum:

Talk to Your Doctor: Before incorporating cranberries into your UTI prevention plan, discuss it with your doctor. They can help you determine if cranberry products might be a suitable option based on your individual health history and UTI risk factors.

Consider the Quality: If you choose to try cranberry products, opt for high-quality options with a good concentration of PACs. Read labels carefully and choose products with minimal added sugars or artificial ingredients.

Don't Rely Solely on Cranberries: Cranberries should not be seen as a magic bullet for UTIs. A comprehensive approach that includes staying hydrated, practicing good hygiene, and addressing underlying risk factors remains crucial for UTI prevention.

## The Future of Cranberries:  Research on the Horizon

The research on cranberries and UTIs is ongoing.  Future studies might shed more light on the effectiveness of various cranberry products, their impact on different populations, and the optimal dosages for UTI prevention.

Cranberries hold potential as a natural UTI prevention strategy, particularly for those with recurrent infections. However, the research is still evolving.  By discussing it with your doctor and incorporating cranberries as part of a multifaceted approach to UTI prevention, you can take charge of your urinary health and keep UTIs at bay.

## 5.2 Beyond Cranberries: Other UTI-Friendly Foods and Supplements

Cranberries might be the poster child for UTI prevention, but they're not the only player on the field. This chapter sift into a wider range of dietary choices and supplements that can promote urinary tract health and potentially reduce your risk of UTIs. Think of it as expanding your UTI prevention toolkit with a variety of tools to keep those pesky infections at bay.

### Dietary Choices for a Healthy Urinary Tract: Power Up Your Plate

Here are some dietary superstars that can contribute to a healthy urinary tract and potentially lower your susceptibility to UTIs:

Hydration Heroes: Water remains the undisputed champion in UTI prevention. Drinking plenty of fluids throughout the day helps dilute urine, preventing bacteria from adhering to the bladder wall and flushing them out efficiently. Aim for eight glasses of water per day, or tailor your intake based on your activity level and climate.

Fiber Fantastic Foods:  Fiber-rich foods play a crucial role in maintaining a healthy digestive system.  A balanced gut microbiome can indirectly support urinary health by boosting your immune system, which helps your body fight off infections.  Fruits, vegetables, whole grains, and legumes are all excellent sources of fiber.

Vitamin C Powerhouse:  Vitamin C is a well-known immune system booster.  Including vitamin C-rich fruits and vegetables in your diet can help keep your body's defenses strong, potentially aiding in preventing UTIs. Think citrus fruits, bell peppers, broccoli, and berries.

Probiotic Power:  Probiotics are live bacteria that offer various health benefits, including promoting a healthy gut microbiome.  Some studies suggest that probiotic-rich foods like yogurt or fermented foods like kimchi might offer some benefit in preventing UTIs.

Important Note:  While these dietary choices can be helpful, they are not guaranteed UTI prevention strategies. Always consult with your doctor before making significant changes to your diet, especially if you have any underlying health conditions.

## Supplements for UTI Prevention: Exploring the Options

Certain supplements might offer some additional support for urinary tract health.  Here's a closer look at some popular options:

- D-Mannose:  This simple sugar has gained popularity in recent years for its potential role in UTI prevention.  D-mannose is thought to work by interfering with the ability of E. coli bacteria to adhere to the bladder wall.  However, research on D-mannose is still ongoing, and its effectiveness might vary from person to person.

- Probiotic Supplements: While probiotic-rich foods can be beneficial, some people might choose to take concentrated probiotic supplements.  These supplements can provide a higher dose of live bacteria and might offer additional support for urinary health.  Again, consult your doctor before starting any new supplements.

**A Word of Caution:  Supplements Aren't Magic Bullets**

It's important to remember that supplements are not a substitute for a healthy lifestyle and evidence-based UTI prevention strategies.  Here are some key points to consider:

Limited Research: The research on many supplements for UTI prevention is still developing. More studies are needed to confirm their long-term efficacy and safety.

Individual Differences: People might respond differently to various supplements. What works for one person might not be effective for another.

Doctor Discussion is Key: Before starting any new supplements, discuss them with your doctor. They can help you determine if supplements are a suitable option for you and ensure they don't interact with any medications you're currently taking.

## A Multifaceted Approach for Optimal Health

A combination of dietary choices, proper hydration, and potentially certain supplements, in consultation with your doctor, can create a holistic approach to promoting urinary tract health and minimizing your risk of UTIs.  Remember, consistency is key.

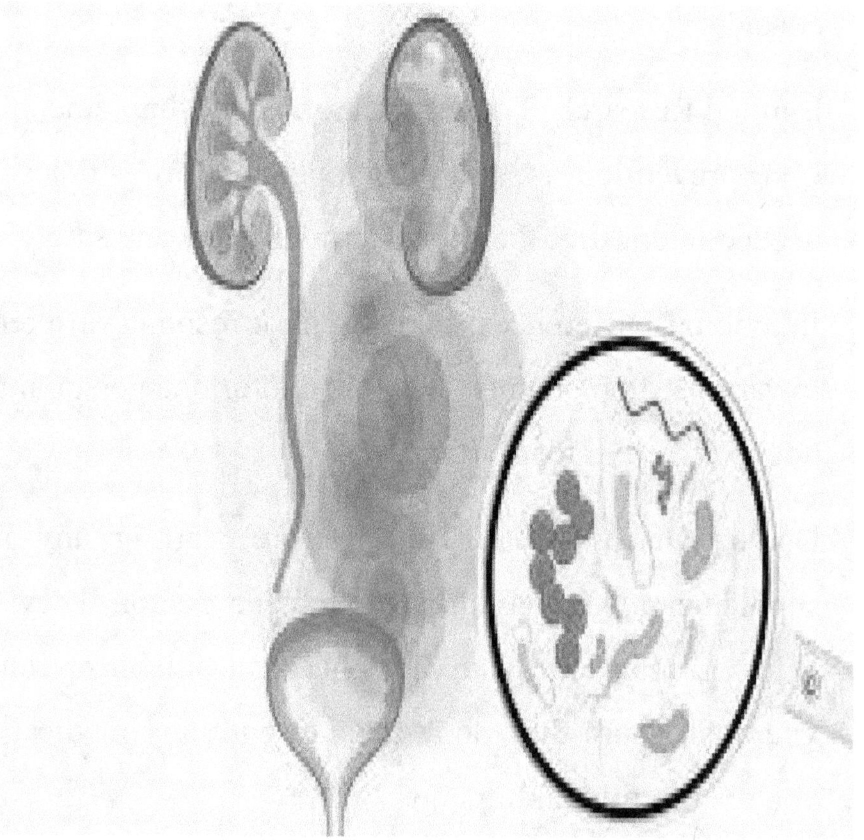

# CHAPTER SIX

## 6.1 COTTON CRUSADERS: DITCHING IRRITATING FABRICS

When it comes to fighting urinary tract infections (UTIs), the battleground often extends beyond just what you ingest. Believe it or not, the type of underwear you wear can play a significant role in your susceptibility to these pesky infections. This chapter go into the science behind fabric choices and unveils why cotton underwear reigns supreme as a UTI prevention champion.

**The Fabric Factor: Understanding the Material Impact**

The material of your underwear directly impacts the environment around your delicate genital area. Here's how fabric choices can influence your UTI risk:

Breathability Matters: Cotton is a natural fiber known for its breathability. It allows air to circulate freely, preventing moisture buildup in the genital area. This moisture control is crucial for preventing the growth of bacteria that can lead to UTIs.

Synthetic Woes: Synthetic fabrics like nylon and spandex, while comfortable and stretchy, often lack breathability. They trap moisture and heat, creating a breeding ground for bacteria. Think of it like a humid greenhouse – perfect for unwanted bacterial growth.

**The Friction Factor:  Comfort Counts**

Beyond breathability, the texture of your underwear fabric also plays a role. Synthetic fabrics can sometimes be rough or irritating, especially on sensitive skin. This friction can further disrupt the natural balance of the vaginal flora and potentially increase susceptibility to UTIs.

Cotton's Comfort Advantage:  Cotton is a soft, gentle fabric that conforms to your body without causing irritation. This comfort factor helps maintain a healthy environment for your genital area, reducing the risk of UTIs.

## Cotton's Additional Benefits

Here are some additional reasons why cotton underwear deserves a starring role in your UTI prevention strategy:

Natural Moisture Absorption: Cotton is naturally absorbent, wicking away moisture from the skin and preventing it from accumulating in the genital area. This helps keep you feeling fresh and dry throughout the day.

Hypoallergenic: Cotton is a hypoallergenic material, making it less likely to irritate sensitive skin. This is particularly important for those prone to skin sensitivities or allergies.

Easy Care: Cotton underwear is generally easy to care for and can be washed and dried at moderate temperatures. This makes it a convenient and practical choice for everyday wear.

**The Synthetic Downside:  Drawbacks to Consider**

While synthetic fabrics might have their advantages in terms of stretch and fit, here are some drawbacks to consider when it comes to UTIs:

Yeast Infection Risk: The warm, moist environment created by synthetic fabrics can also increase the risk of yeast infections. Yeast thrives in these conditions, and UTIs and yeast infections can sometimes co-occur.

Trapped Odors: Synthetic fabrics can trap odors more readily compared to cotton. This can be not only unpleasant but also potentially contribute to irritation.

**Cotton for the Win!**

When it comes to UTI prevention, cotton underwear emerges as the clear victor.  Its breathability, comfort, absorbency, and hypoallergenic properties make it an ideal choice for maintaining a healthy genital environment and minimizing UTI risk.

In coming chapters of this book will explore additional lifestyle strategies and medical interventions for UTIs. By incorporating cotton underwear into your daily routine alongside other preventative measures, you can create a powerful defense system against these infections and maintain optimal urinary tract health. So, ditch the synthetics and embrace the comfort and protection of cotton underwear – your body will thank you!

## 6.2 Stress Less, Flow More: Managing Stress for Bladder Health

Urinary tract infections (UTIs) are often viewed as purely physical ailments, brought on by bacteria and addressed with medication. However, the mind-body connection plays a surprising role in UTI susceptibility. Chronic stress, that unwelcome companion in our modern lives, can actually increase your risk of developing these infections. This chapter examine into the science behind stress and UTIs, and unveils how stress management techniques like yoga and meditation can become powerful allies in your UTI prevention strategy.

## The Stress-UTI Connection: When Your Body Talks Back

Stress is a natural response to challenging situations. It triggers the release of hormones like cortisol, which prepares your body for fight-or-flight scenarios. While this response is crucial for survival in the short term, chronic stress can wreak havoc on your overall health, including your urinary tract.

**Here's how chronic stress can contribute to UTIs:**

Weakened Immune System: Chronic stress can suppress the immune system, making it harder for your body to fight off infections, including those caused by E. coli, the common culprit in UTIs. Think of your immune system as your body's army – chronic stress weakens the troops, leaving them vulnerable to invaders.

Bladder Muscle Spasticity: Stress can lead to muscle tension throughout the body, including the muscles in the bladder. This tension can cause the bladder to become hyperactive or irritable, making it difficult to completely empty the bladder. Remember, stagnant urine becomes a breeding ground for bacteria.

**The Calming Counteroffensive: Stress Management Techniques to the Rescue**

The good news is that by managing stress, you can significantly reduce your risk of UTIs. Here are some powerful stress management techniques that can become your allies in the fight against these infections:

Yoga: This ancient practice combines physical postures, breathing exercises, and meditation. Yoga has been shown to reduce stress hormones, promote relaxation, and improve overall well-being. Regular yoga practice can contribute to a stronger immune system and a healthier urinary tract.

Meditation: Meditation involves focusing your attention and quieting the mind. Regular meditation practice can help reduce stress, improve emotional regulation, and promote a sense of calm. This inner peace can translate to a healthier urinary tract.

Deep Breathing: Simple deep breathing exercises can be a powerful tool for managing stress in the moment. Taking slow, deep breaths activates the relaxation response in your body, counteracting the fight-or-flight response triggered by stress.

**Stress Management for Busy Lives**

While yoga studios and meditation retreats offer a dedicated space for stress management, you can incorporate these techniques into your daily routine, no matter how busy you are:

Start Small: Begin with short yoga sequences or meditation sessions that fit comfortably into your schedule. Even five minutes a day can make a difference.

Mindful Moments: Throughout the day, take a few deep breaths to center yourself and manage stress in the moment. These mindful pauses can interrupt the stress cycle and promote relaxation.

Identify Stressors: Pay attention to what triggers your stress and explore ways to minimize those triggers or develop coping mechanisms. This proactive approach can help you manage stress before it takes a toll on your health.

## Stress Less, UTIs Less

Chronic stress can be a contributing factor to UTIs. By incorporating stress management techniques like yoga, meditation, and deep breathing into your daily routine, you can empower yourself to reduce stress, strengthen your immune system, and create a healthier environment for your urinary tract. Remember, a multifaceted approach that addresses both physical and mental factors is key to winning the battle against UTIs and achieving optimal urinary health. So, take a deep breath, embrace stress management techniques, and take charge of your well-being!

# CHAPTER SEVEN

## 7.1 TESTING THE WATERS: DIAGNOSTIC TECHNIQUES FOR UTIS

Urinary tract infections (UTIs) can be a real drag, causing discomfort and disruption to your daily routine. But before you can conquer them, you need to confirm their presence. This chapter dig into the world of diagnostic tests used by doctors to identify UTIs and pinpoint the specific bacterial culprits. Think of these tests as detective work – gathering evidence to solve the case of the unhappy urinary tract.

**The Diagnostic Do-Si-Do: A Multi-Step Approach**

Diagnosing a UTI typically involves a combination of tests. Here's a closer look at the common diagnostic tools used:

Urine Analysis (Urinalysis): This is often the first step in UTI diagnosis. A urinalysis involves examining a urine sample for abnormalities like:

White Blood Cells (WBCs): An elevated WBC count in the urine can indicate inflammation, a potential sign of infection.

Red Blood Cells (RBCs): The presence of red blood cells might suggest irritation or bleeding in the urinary tract.

Nitrates: Bacteria can break down certain substances in urine, leading to the presence of nitrates. However, a negative nitrate test doesn't necessarily rule out a UTI.

Leukocyte Esterase (LE): The presence of LE, an enzyme produced by white blood cells, can also be an indicator of infection.

Urine Culture: While a urinalysis can provide clues, a urine culture is the gold standard for UTI diagnosis. This test involves collecting a urine sample and letting it grow in a controlled environment. If bacteria are present, they will multiply, allowing doctors to identify the specific type of bacteria causing the infection. This information is crucial for choosing the most effective antibiotic treatment.

## Additional Tests in Special Cases

In some cases, additional tests might be necessary to rule out other conditions or get a clearer picture of the UTI:

- Imaging Tests: X-rays, ultrasounds, or CT scans might be used if there's a concern about structural abnormalities in the urinary tract that might be contributing to UTIs.

- Cystoscopy: This test involves inserting a thin tube with a camera into the bladder to directly visualize the bladder lining and urethra. This is typically used for recurrent UTIs or when there's a suspicion of underlying conditions.

## Decoding the Diagnosis

The results of your diagnostic tests will help your doctor determine the presence or absence of a UTI. Here's a breakdown of what your results might mean:

Positive Urinalysis and Culture: This confirms a UTI, and the bacteria identified in the culture will guide antibiotic selection.

Positive Urinalysis, Negative Culture: This might indicate a non-bacterial UTI or a very low bacterial count. Your doctor will determine the next steps based on your symptoms and medical history.

Negative Urinalysis: This might suggest another cause for your symptoms, and your doctor might order further tests to rule out other conditions.

Diagnostic tests play a crucial role in accurately diagnosing UTIs. By providing valuable information about the presence of bacteria and their types, these tests empower doctors to prescribe the most effective treatment for your specific infection. So, don't hesitate to seek medical evaluation if you suspect a UTI, and let the diagnostic tests help you crack the code and get back to feeling your best!

## 7.2 Antibiotics Aren't Always the Answer: Exploring Treatment Options

Urinary tract infections (UTIs) are no match for a well-armed warrior – you! Armed with the knowledge from the previous chapter about diagnostic tests, you're ready for the next step: treatment. This chapter explores the various weapons in your UTI-fighting arsenal, from the tried-and-true antibiotics to other potential strategies. Think of it as a strategic war room, where you and your doctor decide on the most effective course of action to vanquish the UTI foe.

## The Antibiotic Arsenal: The First Line of Defense

Antibiotics remain the mainstay of UTI treatment. These powerful medications target and kill bacteria, effectively eliminating the infection. Here's a breakdown of some commonly used antibiotics for UTIs:

Trimethoprim-sulfamethoxazole (TMP-SMX): This is a popular first-line antibiotic for uncomplicated UTIs. It's generally well-tolerated and effective against a broad spectrum of bacteria commonly implicated in UTIs.

Nitrofurantoin: Another first-line option, nitrofurantoin is particularly useful for uncomplicated UTIs because it has a lower risk of developing bacterial resistance compared to some other antibiotics.

Cephalosporins: These antibiotics might be used if you're allergic to TMP-SMX or nitrofurantoin, or if the bacteria causing your UTI is resistant to other options.

Fluoroquinolones: These powerful antibiotics are typically reserved for more complex UTIs, such as kidney infections, or in cases where other antibiotics haven't been effective. Fluoroquinolones can have some side effects, so their use is carefully considered.

**Choosing the Right Weapon: Tailoring Treatment to the Infection**

The specific antibiotic chosen for your UTI will depend on several factors:

Type of Bacteria: The urine culture results will identify the specific bacteria causing the infection. This information is crucial for selecting the most effective antibiotic.

Severity of Infection: Uncomplicated bladder infections typically require a shorter course of antibiotics compared to more complex UTIs like kidney infections.

Allergic Reactions: If you have allergies to certain antibiotics, your doctor will choose an alternative that's safe for you.

## Beyond Antibiotics: Exploring Alternative Approaches

While antibiotics are the cornerstone of UTI treatment, there are some additional strategies that might be considered, especially for recurrent UTIs:

Low-Dose Long-Term Antibiotics: In some cases, your doctor might recommend taking a low dose of antibiotics for a longer duration to prevent recurrent UTIs.

Cranberry Products: While research is ongoing, some studies suggest that cranberry juice or cranberry supplements might offer some benefit in preventing UTIs, particularly for women with recurrent infections. However, their effectiveness can vary from person to person.

Important Note:  These alternative approaches should not be used without consulting your doctor.  Antibiotics are still the primary treatment for active UTIs.

Remember, you're not alone in this battle against UTIs. Your doctor will work with you to determine the most effective treatment plan based on your specific infection and medical history.  By following your doctor's instructions for medication use and potentially incorporating lifestyle changes, you can conquer the UTI and reclaim your urinary tract health. So, work closely with your doctor, choose the right weapon for the fight, and get ready to banish the UTI for good!

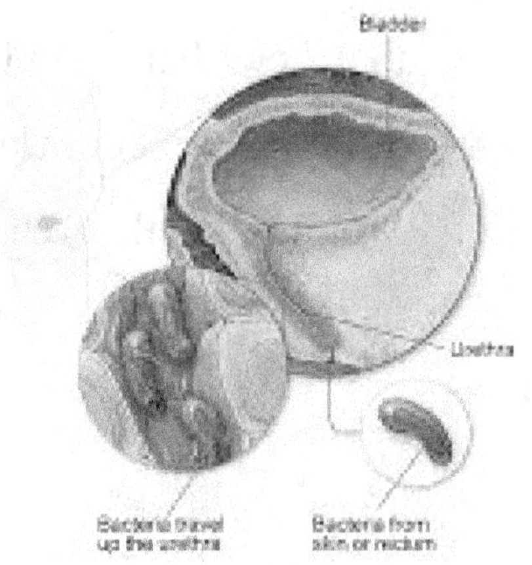

# CHAPTER EIGHT

## 8.1 SOOTHING SOLUTIONS: PAIN RELIEF STRATEGIES

Urinary tract infections (UTIs) can be a real pain – literally. The burning, urgency, and discomfort associated with UTIs can disrupt your daily routine and leave you feeling miserable. While antibiotics are the primary treatment for UTIs, there are also natural remedies that can offer some relief from the unpleasant symptoms. Think of these remedies as gentle warriors in your UTI battle plan, providing comfort and easing the discomfort while the antibiotics do their job of eliminating the infection.

### The Heat is on: Harnessing the Power of Warmth

Heat therapy is a simple yet effective way to ease the pain and discomfort associated with UTIs. Here's how it works:

Relaxing Muscle Tension: UTIs can cause muscle tension in the pelvic floor and bladder. Applying heat helps relax these muscles, reducing the burning sensation and urgency to urinate.

Improved Blood Flow: Heat increases blood flow to the area, which can promote healing and reduce inflammation.

**Natural Heat Therapy Options:**

Heating Pad: A trusty heating pad applied to your lower abdomen can provide localized warmth and significant relief. Use a low to medium heat setting and place a thin towel between the heating pad and your skin to avoid burns.

Warm Bath: Immersing yourself in a warm bath can be a soothing and relaxing way to ease UTI discomfort. Add some Epsom salts to the bath for an extra dose of relaxation. Remember to avoid very hot baths, as they can irritate the skin.

**Hydration Heroes:  Drink Your Way to Relief**

While UTIs might make you feel like avoiding fluids altogether, staying hydrated is crucial for flushing out bacteria and speeding up the healing process.  Here's why:

Dilution is Key: Drinking plenty of fluids dilutes urine, making it less irritating to the bladder lining and reducing the burning sensation.

Frequent Flushes: Increased urination helps flush out bacteria from the urinary tract, preventing them from multiplying and worsening the infection.

**Hydration Options for UTI Relief**

While water is the ultimate hydrator, here are some other options you can incorporate:

Cranberry Juice: While research on cranberry juice for UTI prevention is mixed, some studies suggest it might offer some relief from symptoms. Choose unsweetened cranberry juice with a high concentration of PACs (proanthocyanidins) for potential benefit.

Herbal Teas: Certain herbal teas, like chamomile or peppermint, might have mild anti-inflammatory properties that can provide some comfort. However, speak with your doctor before consuming any herbal remedies, especially if you are taking medications.

**Comforting Companions: Lifestyle Modifications for Relief**

Here are some additional lifestyle changes that can ease the discomfort of UTIs:

Frequent Urination: Don't hold back! Emptying your bladder frequently helps prevent bacteria from accumulating and can reduce the burning sensation.

Pain Relief Medication: Over-the-counter pain relievers like acetaminophen or ibuprofen can help manage the aches and pains associated with UTIs. Always follow the dosage instructions carefully.

Loose-Fitting Clothing: Tight clothing can irritate the bladder and urethra. Opt for loose-fitting, breathable cotton underwear and pants for maximum comfort.

Important Note: These natural remedies are meant to provide comfort alongside medical treatment. Always consult your doctor before starting any new supplements or remedies, especially if you have any underlying health conditions.

While these natural remedies can't cure a UTI on their own, they can be powerful allies in your quest for comfort during the course of an infection. By combining heat therapy, proper hydration, lifestyle modifications, and potentially pain relief medication with your doctor-prescribed antibiotics, you can create a multi-pronged approach to soothe the discomfort and promote healing. So, embrace these natural remedies, prioritize comfort, and work with your doctor to banish the UTI and reclaim your well-being!

## 8.2 Natural Reinforcements: Supporting Your Body's Defenses

Urinary tract infections (UTIs) can feel like unwelcome invaders in your body. While antibiotics are the frontline fighters in this battle, some natural supplements might offer additional support for your immune system, potentially aiding in your body's natural defense against UTIs.  This chapter excavate into the world of these potential allies, exploring the science behind them and their possible role in UTI prevention and recovery.  Think of these supplements as reinforcements for your body's natural defenses, working alongside other strategies to create a stronger defense system against UTIs.

**Important Disclaimer:   Supplements Aren't Magic Bullets**

Before diving in, it's crucial to remember that natural supplements are not a guaranteed solution for preventing or treating UTIs.  Here are some key points to consider:

Limited Research: The research on many supplements and their effectiveness against UTIs is ongoing. More studies are needed to confirm their long-term benefits.

Individual Differences: People might respond differently to various supplements. What works for one person might not be as effective for another.

Doctor Discussion is Key: Always consult your doctor before starting any new supplements. They can help you determine if supplements are a suitable option for you and ensure they don't interact with any medications you're currently taking.

With these disclaimers in mind, let's explore some of the natural supplements that have shown promise in supporting the body's defense against UTIs:

D-Mannose: This simple sugar has gained popularity in recent years for its potential role in UTI prevention. D-mannose is thought to work by interfering with the ability of E. coli bacteria to adhere to the bladder wall. This can prevent them from colonizing and causing infection. However, research results on D-mannose are mixed, and its effectiveness might vary from person to person.

Probiotic Supplements: These supplements contain live bacteria that can help maintain a healthy balance of gut flora. A healthy gut microbiome might indirectly support urinary tract health by boosting your overall immune system. Some studies suggest that specific probiotic strains might offer additional benefits in preventing UTIs, particularly for women with recurrent infections.

Vitamin C:  This well-known immune system booster can potentially help keep your body's defenses strong, potentially aiding in preventing UTIs.  Including vitamin C-rich fruits and vegetables like citrus fruits, bell peppers, and berries in your diet is a great way to increase your intake.

Garlic:  Garlic has been used for centuries for its potential medicinal properties.  Some studies suggest that garlic might have antibacterial effects and could potentially offer some benefit in preventing UTIs.  However, more research is needed to confirm its effectiveness.

Elderberry:  This popular herbal remedy has shown promise in boosting the immune system and fighting off viral infections.  While research on its impact on UTIs is limited, some studies suggest it might offer some benefit. It's important to note that elderberry can interact with certain medications, so consulting your doctor is crucial before using it.

Remember: Supplements should be viewed as complementary to, not a replacement for, a healthy lifestyle and evidence-based UTI prevention strategies. Here are some additional considerations:

Quality Matters: Choose high-quality supplements from reputable brands. Look for third-party certifications that ensure purity and potency.

Dosage Matters: Follow the recommended dosage on the supplement label or as directed by your doctor. More isn't necessarily better when it comes to supplements.

Consistency is Key: For some supplements, like probiotics, consistent use might be necessary to see potential benefits.

While natural supplements might offer some additional support, they are just one piece of the UTI prevention and management puzzle. A combination of dietary choices, proper hydration, potentially certain supplements in consultation with your doctor, and addressing underlying risk factors can create a holistic approach to promoting urinary tract health and minimizing your risk of UTIs. So, consider these natural supplements as potential allies, but remember, a comprehensive approach is key to keeping UTIs at bay!

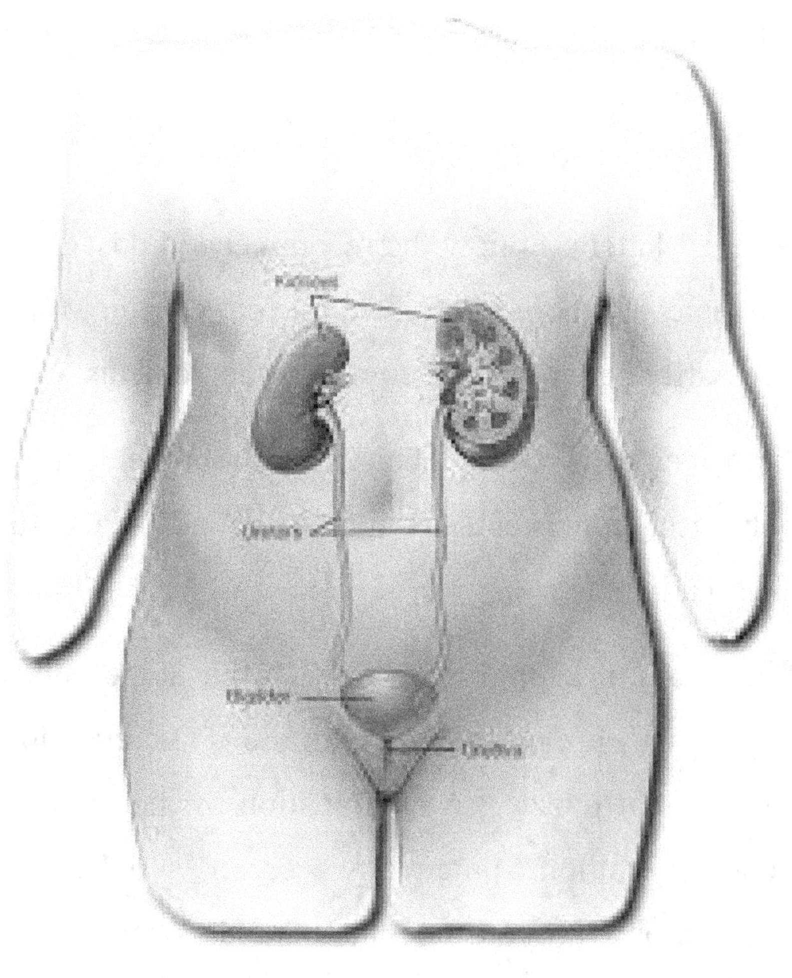

# CHAPTER NINE

## 9.1 IDENTIFYING UNDERLYING CAUSES: WHY DO UTIS KEEP COMING BACK?

Urinary tract infections (UTIs) can be a frustrating foe, especially when they become recurrent visitors. While the typical narrative focuses on battling bacteria, there can be more to the story. This chapter jump into the world of underlying causes that might contribute to recurrent UTIs, empowering you to explore potential explanations beyond just the bacterial culprits. Think of it as detective work – uncovering the root cause of the problem to develop a more effective prevention strategy.

**The Recurrence Riddle: When UTIs Become a Pattern**

While occasional UTIs happen, experiencing them frequently (generally defined as three or more in a year) suggests there might be an underlying reason for their persistence. Here are some potential culprits:

Anatomical Abnormalities: Certain structural issues in the urinary tract can make it easier for bacteria to gain a foothold and cause UTIs. These abnormalities might include:

Urethral Diverticulum: A small pouch in the urethra can trap urine and create a breeding ground for bacteria.

Vesicoureteral Reflux (VUR): A condition where urine flows backward from the bladder to the kidneys, increasing the risk of infection.

Kidney Stones: The presence of stones in the kidneys can obstruct urine flow and create a stagnant environment prone to infection.

Functional Issues: Sometimes, problems with how the bladder or muscles in the urinary tract function can contribute to UTIs. For example:

Neurogenic Bladder: A condition where nerve damage affects bladder function, making it difficult to empty the bladder completely. Residual urine can harbor bacteria.

Overactive Bladder: This condition can lead to frequent urination, potentially pushing bacteria up into the urethra and bladder.

Other Medical Conditions: Certain medical conditions can increase your susceptibility to UTIs, such as diabetes, which can weaken the immune system and make you more prone to infections overall.

## Identifying the Culprit: Diagnostic Tools for Underlying Causes

If you experience recurrent UTIs, your doctor will likely investigate potential underlying causes. Here are some diagnostic tools that might be used:

- Imaging Tests: X-rays, ultrasounds, or CT scans can help visualize the urinary tract and identify any structural abnormalities.

- Urodynamic Testing: This test assesses how well your bladder and urethra store and release urine, revealing any functional issues.

Exploring potential underlying causes of recurrent UTIs is crucial for developing a targeted prevention strategy. By working with your doctor to identify any contributing factors, you can create a more comprehensive approach to keeping UTIs at bay. So, don't hesitate to seek answers beyond the bacteria – uncovering the root cause can be the key to breaking free from the cycle of recurrent UTIs.

## 9.2 Long-Term Strategies: Preventing Recurrent UTIs

Recurrent UTIs can feel like a never-ending battle. Just when you think you've conquered one infection, another one seems to be lurking around the corner. But fear not, warrior! This chapter equips you with an arsenal of strategies to prevent recurrent UTIs, empowering you to take charge of your urinary tract health. Think of it as a war council, where we devise a multi-pronged attack to keep those pesky UTIs at bay.

## Beyond Antibiotics:  A Holistic Approach to Prevention

While antibiotics are crucial for treating UTIs, a holistic approach is key to preventing them from becoming recurrent visitors.  Here are some powerful weapons in your preventative arsenal:

Hydration is King (or Queen):  Drinking plenty of fluids, especially water, is the cornerstone of UTI prevention. Adequate hydration dilutes urine, flushes out bacteria, and keeps your urinary tract healthy.  Aim for eight glasses of water per day, or more if you're active or live in a hot climate.

Wiping Wisdom: Proper wiping technique can make a big difference.  Always wipe from front to back to prevent bacteria from being transferred from the rectum to the urethra.

Frequent Urination: Don't hold it in! Holding urine allows bacteria to multiply in the bladder.  Empty your bladder whenever you feel the urge, and don't ignore that feeling.

Cranberry Power (Maybe):  While research is ongoing, some studies suggest that cranberry products like unsweetened cranberry juice or cranberry supplements might offer some benefit in preventing UTIs, particularly for women with recurrent infections.  However, their effectiveness can vary from person to person.  Discuss this option with your doctor.

Probiotic Powerhouse:  Maintaining a healthy gut microbiome with probiotic supplements might indirectly support urinary tract health by boosting your overall immune system.  Some studies suggest that specific probiotic strains might be particularly helpful in preventing UTIs for those prone to them.  Talk to your doctor about choosing the right probiotic for you.

Post-Intercourse Power Play:  Emptying your bladder after sexual intercourse can help flush out bacteria that might have been introduced during intimacy.

Cotton is King (or Queen) of Underwear:  Ditch the synthetic underwear and opt for breathable cotton options.

Tight-fitting clothing can trap moisture and irritate the urethra, creating a breeding ground for bacteria.

**Long-Term Prophylaxis:  A Doctor's Call**

In some cases, your doctor might recommend a strategy called long-term prophylaxis with low-dose antibiotics. This involves taking a low dose of antibiotics for a prolonged period, typically several months, to prevent UTIs from occurring.  Here's what to consider with this approach:

It's a Doctor's Decision: Long-term antibiotic use should only be done under the guidance of your doctor, as it can contribute to antibiotic resistance.

Not a One-Size-Fits-All Approach: This strategy might not be suitable for everyone. Your doctor will consider your individual situation and weigh the risks and benefits before recommending it.

Preventing recurrent UTIs is a collaborative effort between you and your doctor.  By incorporating these preventative strategies into your daily routine and working with your doctor to address any underlying causes, you can significantly reduce your risk of UTIs and reclaim control of your urinary tract health. So, arm yourself with these preventative strategies, work closely with your doctor, and say goodbye to recurrent UTIs!

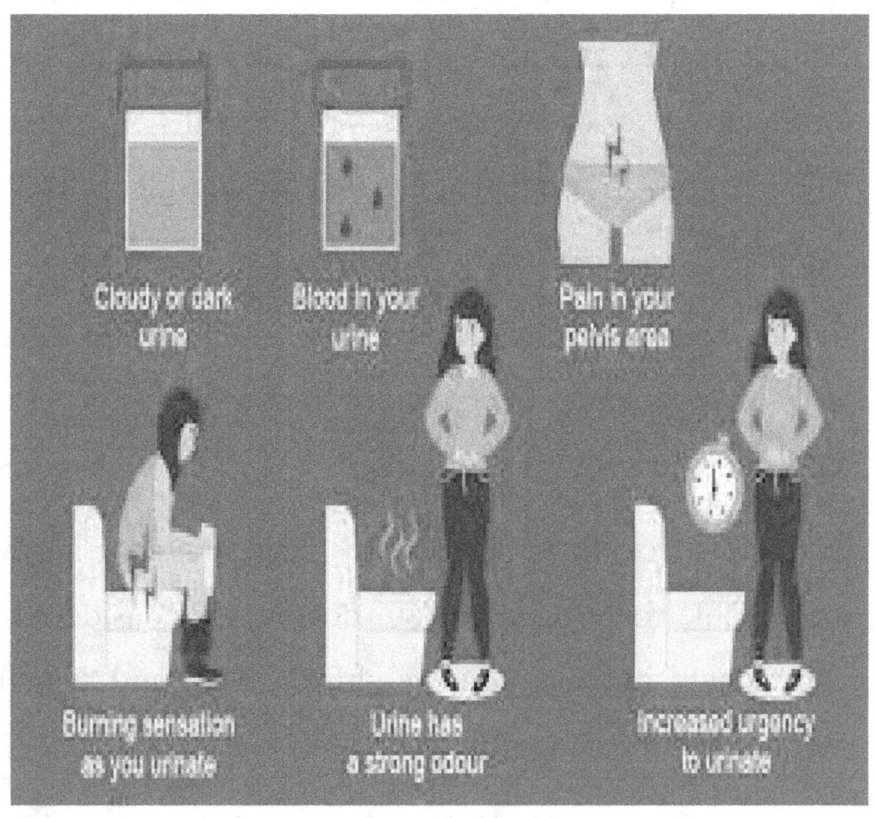

# CHAPTER TEN

## 10.1 YOU ARE NOT ALONE: THE POWER OF COMMUNITY AND SUPPORT

Urinary tract infections (UTIs) can be a lonely battle, leaving you feeling isolated and frustrated. But the truth is, you're far from alone. Millions of people experience UTIs each year, and countless others have successfully navigated the challenges of managing them. This chapter go into the power of community and support, showcasing stories of others who have conquered UTIs and emerged stronger. Think of it as a virtual campfire, where you connect with fellow warriors, share experiences, and gain inspiration on your own UTI management journey.

**Christiana's Story:  From Frustration to Freedom**

Christiana, a busy marketing professional, was plagued by recurrent UTIs. "It felt like every few months, I'd be back at the doctor's office with the same burning sensation and discomfort," she recalls. "It was incredibly disruptive to my life." After exploring various strategies, Christiana discovered that a combination of increased hydration, cranberry supplements, and prioritizing post-workout urination significantly reduced her UTI frequency. "It wasn't a magic bullet," she says, "but by making these changes, I finally feel in control." Christiana's story highlights the importance of personal exploration and finding what works best for your unique situation.

**David's Story:  Men and UTIs – Breaking the Silence**

David, a college athlete, was hesitant to seek help for his UTIs. "I thought UTIs were just a woman's problem," he admits. However, after experiencing persistent symptoms, he finally consulted a doctor. "Learning that men can get UTIs too was a relief," David says. His doctor diagnosed an underlying anatomical abnormality and recommended a minimally invasive surgical procedure to correct it. "Since the surgery, I haven't had a single UTI," David shares. His story emphasizes the importance of breaking down stigmas and seeking medical attention regardless of gender.

## The Power of Online Support Groups

The internet has opened doors to virtual communities, allowing people with UTIs to connect and share experiences. Online support groups provide a safe space to:

Ask questions and get advice: Whether you're seeking tips on managing symptoms or navigating treatment options, online communities offer a wealth of information and support.

Find emotional validation: Knowing you're not alone in your struggles can be incredibly comforting. Sharing your experiences with others who understand can alleviate feelings of isolation.

Discover new strategies: By reading about different approaches others have taken, you might discover new tools or routines to add to your own UTI management arsenal.

Online support groups are not a substitute for professional medical advice. Always consult your doctor for diagnosis and treatment plans.

UTIs can be a frustrating foe, but by embracing a sense of community and support, you can find the strength you need to manage them effectively. Sharing your own story and learning from others can be a powerful source of motivation and inspiration. So, connect with others, share your experiences, and remember, you are a UTI warrior, and you have the power to overcome these challenges!

## 10.2 Taking Control: Managing UTIs with Confidence

Urinary tract infections (UTIs) can leave you feeling like a lone soldier on a battlefield. The burning discomfort, the frequent bathroom trips, and the disruption to your daily routine can make you feel isolated and frustrated. But here's the good news: you're not alone in this fight. Millions of people experience UTIs every year, and countless others have successfully navigated the challenges of managing them. This chapter rummage into the power of building bridges – bridges of support and connection within a community of UTI warriors. Here, you'll find stories of others who have conquered UTIs and emerged stronger, fostering a sense of shared experience and inspiration.

## Lisa's Triumph:  From Discouragement to Discovery

Lisa, a yoga instructor known for her calm demeanor, found herself battling a wave of discouragement after a series of recurrent UTIs. "The constant cycle of antibiotics and discomfort was taking a toll on my well-being," she shares. Determined to find a solution, Lisa embarked on a journey of self-discovery.  She researched natural supplements, consulted a nutritionist, and explored stress management techniques.  "It wasn't easy," Lisa admits, "but by incorporating a daily probiotic, managing stress through yoga nidra meditation, and prioritizing sleep, I've significantly reduced the frequency of UTIs." Lisa's story highlights the importance of a holistic approach and the power of individual exploration in managing UTIs.

**Michael's Journey: Open Communication and Advocacy**

Michael, a software engineer, faced a unique challenge. His chronic UTIs were impacting not just his physical health, but also his professional life due to frequent bathroom breaks. Hesitant at first, Michael decided to have an open conversation with his manager. "To my surprise, he was incredibly supportive," Michael recalls. Together, they developed a flexible work arrangement that allowed him to manage his UTIs without jeopardizing his work. Michael's story emphasizes the importance of open communication and self-advocacy. By speaking up about his condition, he found understanding and support within his professional circle.

**Building Your Support System: Resources Beyond the Doctor's Office**

While medical professionals play a crucial role in UTI management, there are additional resources available to build your support system:

Online Support Groups: The internet has fostered vibrant online communities specifically for people with UTIs. These groups offer a safe space to connect with others who understand your struggles, share experiences, and exchange tips on managing symptoms and preventing recurrence.

UTI Advocacy Organizations: Several organizations advocate for research, education, and support for people with UTIs. These organizations can provide valuable resources, connect you with support groups, and empower you to become your own health advocate.

While online support groups offer camaraderie and insights, they shouldn't replace professional medical advice. Always consult your doctor for diagnosis and treatment plans.

UTIs can be a formidable foe, but by fostering a sense of community and reaching out for support, you can find the strength and knowledge to manage them effectively. Sharing your own story and learning from the experiences of others can be a powerful source of motivation and inspiration. So, build bridges of support, connect with others, and remember, you are a UTI warrior, and together, this community can overcome these challenges!

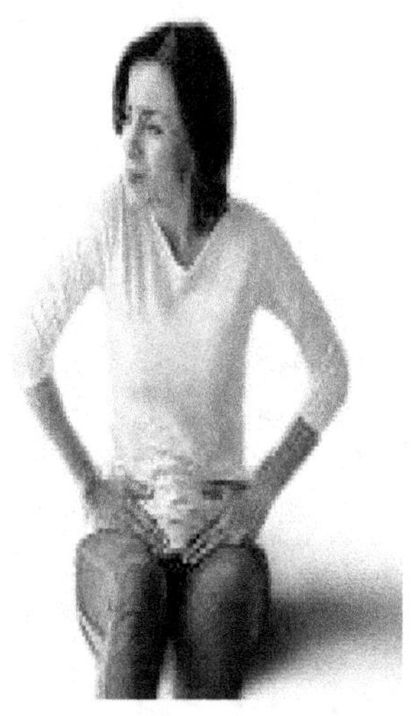

# CHAPTER ELEVEN

## 11.1 KEGELS FOR A STRONGER CORE: EXERCISES FOR BLADDER HEALTH

Urinary tract infections (UTIs) can be a nuisance, but did you know that strengthening your pelvic floor muscles can be a powerful ally in preventing them and improving overall urinary tract health? This chapter dives into the world of Kegel exercises, exploring how these simple yet effective exercises can empower you to take control of your bladder function. Think of your pelvic floor muscles as a hidden hammock supporting your bladder, urethra, and other organs. By strengthening this hammock with Kegel exercises, you can improve bladder control and potentially reduce your risk of UTIs.

**The Pelvic Floor: The Unsung Hero of Urinary Health**

The pelvic floor is a group of muscles that stretches like a sling from the pubic bone to the tailbone. These unsung heroes play a crucial role in various bodily functions, including:

Bladder Control: Strong pelvic floor muscles help hold urine in your bladder and prevent involuntary leakage.

Urinary Flow: These muscles also contribute to complete bladder emptying, preventing residual urine that can harbor bacteria and increase UTI risk.

Sexual Function: Pelvic floor strength can enhance sexual function for both men and women.

**How UTIs Weaken the Pelvic Floor:**

UTIs can actually weaken the pelvic floor muscles. The inflammation and irritation associated with UTIs can cause these muscles to go into spasm or become weak. Weak pelvic floor muscles can contribute to:

- Stress Incontinence: Leaking urine with coughing, sneezing, or laughing.
- Urgency: A sudden, strong urge to urinate that's difficult to control.

- Incomplete Bladder Emptying: Residual urine in the bladder, which can increase UTI risk.

**Enter Kegel Exercises: Your Pelvic Floor's Personal Trainers**

Kegel exercises are simple contractions of the pelvic floor muscles. Think of them as tiny internal weight lifts, strengthening your pelvic floor and improving its function. Here's how to get started:

Find the Muscles: While you can try stopping your urine flow midstream to identify the pelvic floor muscles, this isn't recommended for regular practice. A better approach is to imagine you're trying to hold back gas. The muscles you use for that are your pelvic floor muscles.

Contract and Relax: Tighten your pelvic floor muscles as if you're pulling them upwards. Hold for a count of three, then relax completely for a count of three.

Repeat and Build: Aim for three sets of 10 repetitions daily. As you get stronger, you can gradually increase the hold time and the number of repetitions.

## Kegel Tips for Success

Here are some additional tips to maximize the effectiveness of your Kegel routine:

Focus on Quality, Not Quantity: Focus on squeezing the correct muscles rather than doing a large number of repetitions with improper form.

Consistency is Key: Like any exercise program, consistency is crucial for seeing results. Aim to do your Kegels daily, even if it's just for a few minutes.

Breathe Easy: Don't hold your breath during Kegels. Breathe normally throughout the exercise.

Relax the Rest: Make sure you're only tightening the pelvic floor muscles and not tensing your abdominal muscles, buttocks, or thighs.

Seek Professional Guidance: If you have difficulty performing Kegels or experience any pain, consult a physical therapist specializing in pelvic floor health. They can provide personalized instruction and ensure you're doing the exercises correctly.

Kegel exercises are a simple yet powerful tool for strengthening your pelvic floor muscles and improving bladder control. By incorporating them into your daily routine, you can potentially reduce your risk of UTIs, experience fewer leaks, and gain a greater sense of control over your urinary tract health. So, embrace Kegels, strengthen your pelvic floor, and take charge of your bladder health!

## 11.2 Keeping it Clean: Maintaining Genital Hygiene

Urinary tract infections (UTIs) can be a real drag, interrupting your day with discomfort and urgency. While we've explored various strategies to combat them, prevention is always the best medicine. This chapter dredge into the world of proper genital hygiene practices, equipping you with the knowledge to minimize your risk of UTIs and keep your urinary tract happy. Think of these practices as your personal hygiene superheroes, working tirelessly behind the scenes to prevent unwanted bacterial invaders.

## The Delicate Balance: Maintaining a Healthy Microbiome

The genital area, like other parts of your body, has a delicate microbiome – a community of good and bad bacteria. Maintaining a healthy balance in this microbiome is crucial for preventing UTIs. Here's how proper hygiene practices can help:

Preventing Bad Bacteria Growth: Regular cleaning removes excess sweat, dead skin cells, and potentially harmful bacteria that can irritate the urethra and increase UTI risk.

Keeping Good Bacteria Thriving: Harsh soaps or douching can disrupt the balance of the microbiome, eliminating not just bad bacteria, but also the good bacteria that help keep them in check.

## The Hygiene Heroes: Essential Practices for UTI Prevention

Here are some key genital hygiene practices to incorporate into your daily routine:

Gentle Cleansing: Wash the vulva (the external area) daily with warm water and a mild, fragrance-free cleanser. Avoid harsh soaps or douches, which can irritate the delicate skin and disrupt the natural balance of bacteria.

Wiping Wisdom: Always wipe from front to back after using the toilet. This helps prevent bacteria from the rectum from entering the urethra, which can lead to UTIs. Use soft, unscented toilet paper or wipes.

Cotton Crusaders: Ditch synthetic underwear in favor of breathable cotton options. Cotton allows for better air circulation and prevents moisture buildup, which can create a breeding ground for bacteria.

Post-Play Power Play: Empty your bladder after sexual intercourse. This helps flush out any bacteria that might have been introduced during intimacy.

Listen to Your Body: Change out of sweaty clothes, particularly swimwear, as soon as possible. Moisture can trap bacteria and increase UTI risk.

## Going Beyond the Basics: Additional Tips for Sensitive Skin

If you have sensitive skin, here are some additional tips:

Skip the Douching: Douching is not recommended for anyone, but especially for those with sensitive skin. It can disrupt the natural balance of bacteria and irritate the vaginal lining.

Beware of Scented Products: Avoid soaps, lotions, or wipes with added fragrances, which can irritate the delicate skin in the genital area.

Pat, Don't Rub: When drying the genital area, pat it dry gently with a soft towel instead of rubbing.

When in Doubt, Consult Your Doctor: If you experience any persistent itching, burning, or irritation in the genital area, consult your doctor to rule out any underlying conditions.

By incorporating these simple yet effective genital hygiene practices into your daily routine, you can create a barrier against UTIs and promote overall urinary tract health. Remember, consistency is key! Make these hygiene habits a regular part of your self-care routine, and empower yourself to prevent UTIs before they start. The next chapter of this book will explore additional lifestyle strategies to keep your urinary tract healthy and functioning optimally.

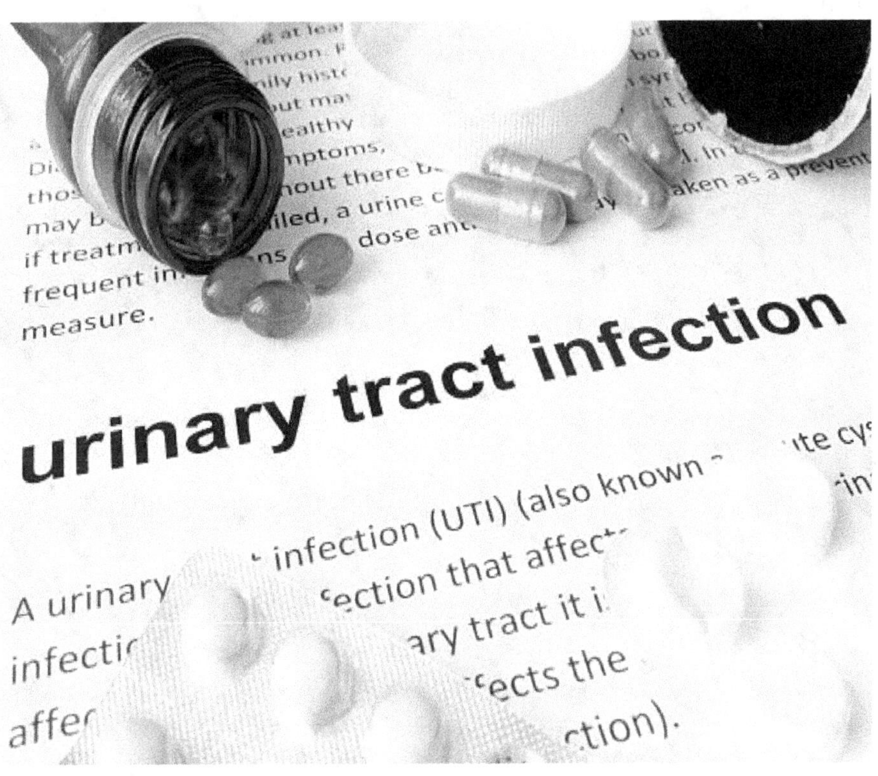

# CHAPTER TWELVE

## 12.1 FINDING THE RIGHT DOCTOR: CHOOSING A UROLOGIST

Urinary tract infections (UTIs) can be frustrating and disruptive, especially if they become recurrent visitors. While managing UTIs often involves lifestyle changes and self-care strategies, sometimes consulting a urologist becomes necessary. This chapter equips you with the knowledge to find a qualified urologist who specializes in urinary tract health, ensuring you partner with the right champion on your journey to optimal urinary health. Think of this as your guide to assembling your UTI dream team – a urologist who listens to your concerns, offers personalized treatment plans, and empowers you to take control of your health.

**What Makes a Urologist a UTI Specialist?**

Urologists are medical doctors who specialize in the urinary tract system, including the kidneys, ureters, bladder, and urethra. While all urologists are qualified to treat UTIs, some have additional training and experience specifically focused on urinary tract health. Here's what to look for in a UTI specialist:

Fellowship Training: Look for urologists who have completed a fellowship in urologic female pelvic medicine and reconstructive surgery (FPMRS). This fellowship provides them with advanced training in conditions that can contribute to recurrent UTIs, such as pelvic floor dysfunction or anatomical abnormalities.

Experience with Recurrent UTIs: Seek a urologist who has experience diagnosing and treating recurrent UTIs. Experience allows them to identify potential underlying causes and develop personalized treatment strategies.

Patient Reviews and Recommendations: Reading online reviews and talking to your primary care physician or friends who have seen a urologist can provide valuable insights into a doctor's bedside manner, communication style, and effectiveness in treating UTIs.

**The Search Begins: Unveiling Your UTI Champion**

Once you know what you're looking for, here are some resources to help you find a qualified urologist:

American Urological Association (AUA): The AUA website allows you to search for urologists in your area based on location, insurance, and areas of expertise. Look for urologists who list "Female Pelvic Medicine and Reconstructive Surgery" among their specialties.

Your Primary Care Physician: Your primary care physician can be a valuable resource for recommendations. They might be familiar with urologists in your area and can provide insights based on your medical history.

Hospital Affiliations: Many hospitals have urology departments. Visiting their website or calling their information line can connect you with urologists on staff.

## The First Consultation: Building a Partnership for UTI Management

When scheduling your first consultation with a urologist, come prepared to discuss your UTI history in detail. Here's what to bring and what to expect:

- Your Medical History: Gather any relevant medical records, including prior UTI test results and medications you're currently taking.

- A List of Questions: Don't hesitate to ask questions about your diagnosis, treatment options, and potential risks and benefits of different approaches.

- An Open Mind and Collaborative Spirit: Think of this consultation as the beginning of a partnership. The best urologists listen to your concerns, involve you in decision-making, and tailor treatment plans to your specific needs and preferences.

Finding the right urologist is crucial for effective UTI management. By looking for specialists with the right qualifications and experience, utilizing available resources, and approaching your first consultation as a collaborative effort, you can assemble your UTI dream team. So, take charge, find your UTI champion, and work together to achieve optimal urinary health!

## 12.2 Staying Informed: Reliable Resources for UTI Information

Urinary tract infections (UTIs) can be a source of frustration and confusion. With so much information available online, it can be challenging to discern reliable sources from myths and misinformation. This chapter equips you with the tools to become an informed patient, empowering you to stay up-to-date on the latest UTI research and treatment options. Think of it as building your own UTI knowledge library, filled with trustworthy resources that can guide you on your journey to optimal urinary tract health.

### Beyond Google: Trustworthy Websites for UTI Information

The internet can be a valuable resource for UTI information, but it's crucial to choose reputable sources. Here are some websites you can trust:

National Institutes of Health (NIH): The NIH website provides a wealth of information on UTIs, including causes, symptoms, diagnosis, and treatment options. Look for the National Institute of Diabetes and Digestive and Kidney Diseases (NIDDK) section on UTIs.

American Urological Association (AUA): The AUA website offers patient education resources on UTIs, including detailed explanations of the urinary tract system, different types of UTIs, and treatment approaches.

Office on Women's Health (OWH): Part of the U.S. Department of Health and Human Services, the OWH website provides information on UTIs specifically for women, addressing common concerns and offering prevention tips.

**Reliable Medical Journals (with a caveat):**

Medical journals contain the latest research findings on UTIs. However, these resources are typically written for healthcare professionals and can be quite technical. If you're interested in exploring medical journals, consider:

Urology: A peer-reviewed journal that publishes original research on various urologic conditions, including UTIs.

The Journal of Urology: Another respected peer-reviewed journal featuring the latest research in urology.

While medical journals offer valuable insights, it's important to discuss any research findings you encounter with your doctor. They can help you interpret the information in the context of your individual situation.

**UTI Support Organizations: A Community of Shared Knowledge**

Several organizations provide support and information for people with UTIs. These organizations can be a great resource for:

Learning about the latest research: Many organizations stay updated on research developments and share them with their members.

Connecting with others: Online forums and support groups can connect you with others who understand your struggles and can share personal experiences and tips.

**Here are some reputable UTI support organizations:**

The Interstitial Cystitis Association (ICA): While their primary focus is on interstitial cystitis (IC), the ICA also offers information on UTIs and related conditions.

The National Association for Continence (NAFC): The NAFC provides resources on various urinary tract issues, including UTIs.

By utilizing these reliable resources, you can become an informed patient, actively participating in your UTI management. Don't hesitate to ask your doctor questions about research findings or treatment options you encounter. The more you know, the better equipped you are to make informed decisions about your health. The final chapter of this book will offer some concluding thoughts and empower you to take charge of your urinary tract health with confidence. So, explore these resources, build your knowledge library, and become an active participant in your UTI management journey!

# GLOSSARY

Antibiotics: Medications that kill or stop the growth of bacteria. They are commonly used to treat UTIs caused by bacterial infections.

Bladder: A muscular sac-like organ that stores urine until it is released from the body through urination.

Cranberry: A fruit sometimes used as a natural remedy to prevent UTIs. Research on its effectiveness is ongoing.

Incomplete Bladder Emptying: When urine remains in the bladder after urination, which can increase the risk of UTIs.

Kegel Exercises: Exercises that strengthen the pelvic floor muscles, which can improve bladder control and potentially reduce UTI risk.

Microbiome: A community of microorganisms, including bacteria, that live in various parts of the body, including the genital area. Maintaining a healthy balance in the microbiome is crucial for preventing UTIs.

Pelvic Floor Muscles: A group of muscles that support the bladder, urethra, uterus (in women), and rectum. Strong pelvic floor muscles contribute to better bladder control.

Probiotics: Live bacteria that are similar to the beneficial bacteria found in the gut. Some studies suggest probiotics might help prevent UTIs.

Recurrent UTIs: Having UTIs that happen frequently, typically defined as two or more UTIs within six months.

Stress Incontinence: Leaking urine due to coughing, sneezing, laughing, or physical activity.

Urgency: A sudden, strong urge to urinate that's difficult to control.

Urethra: The tube that carries urine from the bladder to outside the body.

Urinary Tract: The system that removes waste products from the body in the form of urine. It includes the kidneys, ureters, bladder, and urethra.

Urinary Tract Infection (UTI): An infection in any part of the urinary tract, most commonly caused by bacteria entering the urethra and traveling to the bladder.

Urologist: A doctor who specializes in the urinary tract system and its disorders, including UTIs.

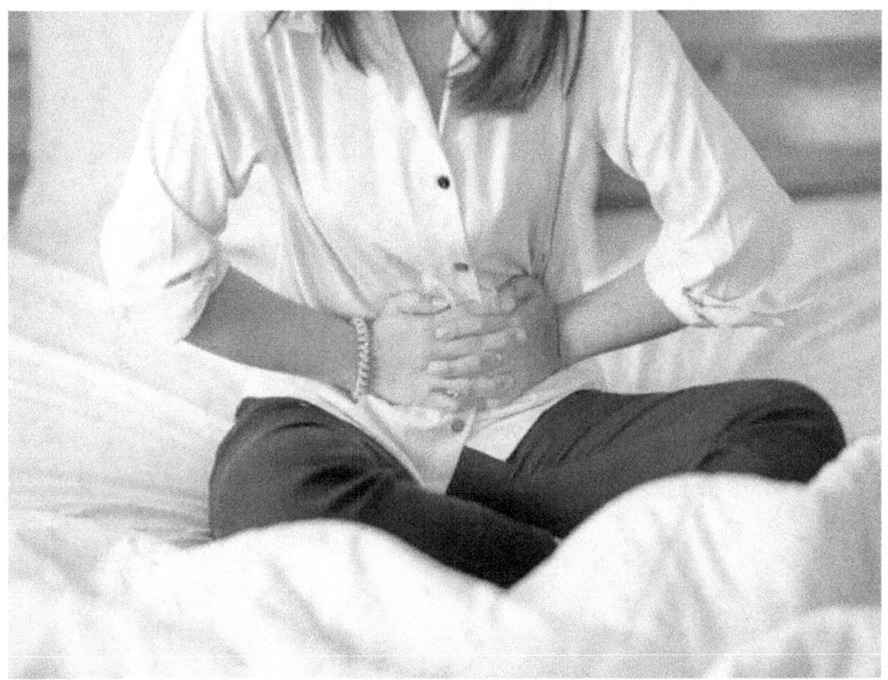

# CONCLUSION

**"The human body is an amazing machine," said Leonardo da Vinci, the renowned scientist and artist.**

And within this machine, the urinary tract plays a vital role, ensuring the removal of waste products and keeping us healthy. But UTIs can throw a wrench into this smooth operation, causing discomfort, disruption, and frustration.

**This book, UTI Decoded: Solutions for a Stress-Free Flow**, has equipped you with the knowledge and tools to combat UTIs and take charge of your urinary tract health. We've dig into the why, the how, and the what-now of UTIs, exploring the causes, prevention strategies, and treatment options. You've learned about strengthening your pelvic floor with Kegel exercises, maintaining a healthy balance with proper hygiene practices, and the importance of partnering with a qualified urologist if needed.

Remember, knowledge is power.  By becoming an informed patient, you can actively participate in your UTI management journey.  Don't be afraid to ask questions, explore reliable resources, and advocate for your own well-being.  The final message? You are not alone in this. Millions of people experience UTIs, and countless others have successfully managed them.  Embrace the strategies outlined in this book, and remember, you have the power to prevent UTIs, manage them effectively, and achieve a stress-free flow.

So, take a deep breath, release any lingering anxieties, and empower yourself with the knowledge you now possess. You are the master of your flow, and with the right tools and strategies, UTIs won't hold you back.  Go forth, live your life, and let your urinary tract health be a source of confidence, not frustration.